Morning Routine
to Wake Up Successful

*Learn to Start your Day with Motivation and
Energy to Upgrade Your Life Forever!*

2nd Edition

Jacky Naismith

information is without contract or any type of guarantee assurance.

The trademarks that are used are without any consent, and the publication of the trademark is without permission or backing by the trademark owner. All trademarks and brands within this book are for clarifying purposes only and are the owned by the owners themselves, not affiliated with this document.

Table of Content

Introduction

Most people who don't already have a morning ritual get up at different times in the morning and they feel sluggish for hours after they're out of bed. That's one reason to start having a morning ritual, but did you know there are others?

A morning ritual actually gives you a reason to get out of your bed rather than lie in bed for half an hour as you stare at the ceiling or catch up on sleep. It also becomes a habit so that you get out of bed at a regular time. That will leave you feeling refreshed and awake all in and of itself. You'll also be starting the day off on the right foot rather than feeling sluggish and slow until well past lunchtime by doing some exercises and eating a healthy breakfast.

If you have a morning ritual, you will feel less rushed and you'll be more relaxed as you're getting ready and heading off to work or school. You'll be giving yourself the needed time to get your mindset right and your body awake. And most importantly, your morning ritual is all about you! You get to spend the needed amount of time every morning in order to center your mind and get your body healthy.

So let's get started with Chapter One: A Good Morning Starts with a Good Night.

Chapter One:
A Good Morning Starts with a Good Night

When people think of a good morning routine, they start by thinking about the moment they open their eyes to the sound of their alarm clock. In all reality, you cannot have a good morning routine without first having a good night's rest. So let's talk about a good nightly routine in order to get you into the habit of getting up when your alarm clock goes off the next morning.

Go to Bed When You're Tired and Wake-up at the Same Time Every Day

First and foremost, never go to bed unless you are actually tired. If you do this, you will mess up your internal clock and you'll never be able to get up on time in the morning. The second thing to do is to make sure you set your alarm clock at the same time every morning, including weekends. Your body will adjust within a matter of days; although, it will take thirty days before you can get up without the alarm clock. When your body has adjusted, it will tell you when it's time for bed at night.

Write down Three Things You're Proud Of

Before you go to bed, you should have a journal where you keep your affirmations for the morning and your good deeds from the day before. Write down three things that you did during the day that you're proud of such as coming up with a great idea at work or just holding the door for someone behind you. It doesn't matter how small the deed may seem, just write it down. Out of the worst day of your life, you will still be able to find three good things that happened. This will give you a positive mindset for the next morning.

Make Time for Family

If you have children, pick a specific time every night that you read them a bedtime story, and be sure to teach them good habits too, such as taking a bath at the same time, brushing their teeth at the same time, and having their bedtime story read to them at the same time. This creates a routine for both you and your children. In addition, be sure to ask them about their day and include them in your evening conversations in order for them to feel as if they're part of the family.

When it comes to your spouse, ask them about their day and talk about relaxing subjects. Avoid hot topics such as politics or religion, and don't bring up any arguments the two of you may have had. Leave those for another time.

Turn off Electronics

Melatonin is the neurotransmitter that prompts us to sleep, and when you have bright lights such as a cell phone or tablet screen directly in front of you as you're attempting to fall asleep, it will take a lot longer because the melatonin will not be released. Therefore, you should turn off all electronics sixty minutes before your planned bedtime. This will prompt you to fall asleep a lot quicker. In addition, turn all your lights down low rather than keeping bedtime lamps burning bright.

Set a Timer to Remind You to Sleep

Just like you set a timer to wake up, set one on your phone to tell you that it's time to shut your electronics off and to turn down your lights. This will help you keep a routine when you're going to bed.

Straighten Up

By putting items back in the place where they belong, you will feel much better about going to bed. Plus, you won't have to worry about doing that in the morning, which will leave you more time to get your morning routine packed full of energizing steps!

Prepare for Morning

If your kids' lunches can be prepared the night before, then do it. If you can set up your breakfast the night before, then get it prepared. There are a lot of things you can do the night before in order to set-up for your routine in the morning.

Practice Mindfulness

There's one simple way to make your mind relax, and that's to relax your body, too. Try a simple mindfulness meditation trick known as the body scan. To do this, you simply lie down in bed on your back. Then tense your right foot and release it. Do the same with your left, and continue up your body until you've tensed your face and relaxed. You should feel the blood flowing through your limbs and your mind should be focused on how relaxed you feel.

Take a Warm Bath

Taking a warm bath was something you did at night in order to get ready for bed when you were a child, but you can do it as an adult too. You don't have to wash your hair if you're going to shower in the morning, but you can submerge your body in the warm water and think about some of the positive things that happened to you that day. Brush your teeth when you get out so that you have a clean feeling when you wake up in the morning.

Drink a Glass of Warm Milk or Herbal Tea

Warm milk has the same amino acid in it known as tryptophan that turkey does, and it's the reason everyone is sleepy after a turkey dinner. Warming up a mug of milk in the microwave for thirty seconds and sipping it will make you feel sleepy within fifteen minutes. It's also a great way to hydrate yourself before bedtime so that you don't wake up thirsty in the middle of the night if it's wintertime.

In addition to milk, herbal, decaffeinated teas are a great way to stay hydrated and they cut out the craving for a cup of coffee or a glass of soda before bed, both of which are caffeinated. Caffeine is one of the main reasons most people are not able to get to sleep at night. In fact, cut off your caffeine consumption by three in the afternoon in order to be caffeine free by the time you want to go to bed.

What to do if you are not sleeping well

As we just talked about getting a good night's rest is vital for a morning routine, but sometimes no matter what we might try before going to bed we find it hard to sleep well. In order for you to be productive and energetic during the day it is important to make sure you sleep well. So, what happens if creating a normal bed time, taking a warm bath to help relax, or even shutting off all electronics at night doesn't help you get the rest that you need? Luckily, there are other things that you can try to help your body get the rest that it requires night after night. And even if you do try out some of these other ideas, it is still a good idea to follow the advice that we gave you above, as those will also help in the long run.

Regular Sleep Schedule

One of the best things that you can do to help get the rest you need each night is to get into a regular sleep schedule. And as long as you stay consistent with your sleep schedule you will benefit greatly in terms of feeling more refreshed and energized. To do this you are going to need to get in touch with your body's natural sleep cycle.

Getting in touch with your natural sleep cycle is going to require a period of about two weeks and some experimenting. The key to finding your natural sleep cycle is going to bed at the same time every night and letting yourself wake up naturally, no getting up with an alarm clock. For people that were sleep deprived before it can take a bit for your body to catch up with your natural cycle, but it is totally worth it in the end. After about two weeks you will find the sleep cycle that works best for you.

Sometimes you have to get up earlier than you want to or you end up staying up later than you should. When this happens you will often find yourself kind of dragging the next day, but no matter what you do don't sleep in. Instead set aside some time later on in the day where you can take a nap. Taking a nap will allow you to stick with your regular sleep schedule; throwing it off by sleeping in can take days to recover from. Just be smart about napping, if it keeps you up too late give it up and always limit your naps to 30 minutes or less.

One of the hardest parts about adopting a regular sleep schedule is fighting off that after dinner tiredness. Many of us tend to sit back and relax once dinner is done and more often than not you find yourself nodding off. If this happens to you, do not give into the urge to take a nap or go to bed early. Instead what you need to do is get up and get your blood moving, so you can make it to your normal bedtime. If you give in and go to bed too early, you have a higher chance of waking up in the middle of the night and not going back to sleep.

Naturally Regulate Your Sleep Cycle

as we mentioned earlier melatonin is the hormone that regulates your sleep cycle. Your body produces melatonin based on light exposure. As the light starts to get darker your body produces more melatonin to help you relax and drift off to sleep. As light gets brighter your body produces less to allow you to stay awake at night. The problem that many of us face with our natural sleep cycle is that artificial light throws off how much melatonin our body is producing, so we might find ourselves more tired during the day and wide awake at night.

Luckily, there are several things you can do to help naturally regulate your sleep cycle. One thing that you need to do is try and increase the amount of light you are exposed to during the day. This can be done by a number of things, including:

- Taking off your sunglasses when you step outside so you can actually feel the light on your face. The light will lower your body's melatonin production so you will feel alert.
- Spending as much time as possible outside during the daytime hours. Each time you get a break at work, step outside and let the sun shine down on you. You can also spend more time outside during the day when you are home, things you normally do in the evening can be done during daylight hours instead.
- Letting the light in. We get it; you have to work in order to survive, which means you have to deal with artificial light. However, that doesn't mean you can't let in

natural light as well. Open up all of the blinds and curtains that you can during the day to let the sun in. You can also relocate your desk, if possible, so that it is closer to the window.

- Using a light therapy box, which should only be done if all else fails. Plus they make a great addition during the winter when the hours of daylight are drastically limited.

Another part of regulating your sleep cycle is to ensure your body is producing melatonin at the right time, which for majority of us is during the evening hours. If you have a hard time settling down at night there are some things that you can do to increase the amount of melatonin your body is producing, including:

- Turn off TV and computer. Several people use their TVs as a way to fall asleep at night, but this is actually counterproductive as the light the TV and computer emits decreases your body's melatonin production. Instead of the TV or computer, simply read a book or listen to music.
- Avoid using electronic readers at night if you are going to read. Electronic readers that have a backlit, the ones that allow you to read them without an additional light source, cause the same problem with melatonin production that TVs and computers do. If you must use an electronic reader find one that requires a separate light source.
- Use low watt light bulbs in your bedroom, especially with any lamps by your bed. The bright light bulbs tell your body it is daytime, so your body will not produce as much melatonin if they are on.

- Use minimal light if you wake up in the middle of the night. If possible try and navigate without any extra light source and do not turn on any lights. Simply do what you need to do and go straight back to bed.
- Keep the room as dark as possible when it is time to sleep. If your blinds let light in consider purchasing some room darkening curtains, they are a heavy duty material that prevents most outside light from coming in. Electrical displays should be covered or faced away from you. The darker the room the better you will sleep at night.

Keeping your bedroom sleep friendly

Your bedroom is the most important room when it comes to sleep, so you need to treat it as such. One of the most important things you can do to your bedroom is to reserve it strictly for sleeping, and a few other activities. What you need to avoid is sitting in your bed and doing stressful or engaging activities, such as work or puzzles. The reason behind this is that using your bed for these kinds of activities engages your mind. This can cause problems at night when you go to relax and go to sleep because your body will think its time to work or play. Reserving it for restful activities, such as sleep, sends your mind a powerful message each time you get into bed.

How you keep your bedroom will also play a role in how well you sleep at night. You want to make sure you keep the noise level down inside your room, as well as keeping your room at a comfortable temperature. Sometimes keeping the noise level down is outside of your control, such as barking dogs or traffic. If that is the case use white noise to help mask the noise. Rooms that are too hot or too cold cause sleep problems; keep your room at a comfortable temperature and provide plenty of ventilation, which fans are great at helping with both.

The last part of your room that you need to look at is your bed. You want to make sure that your bed is comfortable for you, plus you want to make sure it is the right size. Size wise you should be able to fully stretch out on your bed, as well as be able to easily turn over. You shouldn't wake up with a stiff neck or even a backache. If you are, try switching out your pillow or adding more or less support to your bed. Egg crates are a great way to add some extra cushion to a super firm mattress, foam toppers work well too. If all else fails and your mattress is still uncomfortable, you will need to invest in a new one.

Eating right and exercise help with a good night's sleep

It seems that no matter what you are doing, eating right and exercising plays a big role in improving your life. And, if you take a few minutes to think about it, that actually makes sense. The food that you eat fuels your body, while regular exercise ensures your body is functioning like it's supposed too. So with this in mind it shouldn't be a big surprise that eating right and exercising can help you get the sleep you need each night.

One of the biggest issues people face with eating right is not eating at night before going to bed. For many people it seems they get a snack attack just as they are about to crawl into bed. If this happens to you your best bet is to give into the attack, but do so in a controlled manner. Don't gorge yourself on a bunch of junk. Instead eat a small snack that will fill you up and help you rest, such as a half a turkey sandwich or a banana.

The worst thing you can do is eat a big meal right before bed. Instead try making dinner time earlier in the evening. Avoiding the big meal right before bed is important because it takes a lot of work to digest food, which can keep you awake longer at night. Not to mention certain foods can trigger stomach problems, leading to broken sleep. Night caps are something else that should be avoided, as alcohol doesn't help you sleep better as it negatively affects your quality of sleep.

Cutting back on how much you are drinking at night, as well as how much caffeine you are consuming can also help improve your quality of sleep. You might be surprised to learn that caffeine can cause issues up to 12 hours after your last drink, so if you are having sleeping problems you might want to try eliminating it. Drinking too much at night affects sleep quality because you are waking up every so often to go to the bathroom.

Putting yourself back to sleep

Let's be honest here at some point in your life you have woken up in the middle of the night and had a difficult time falling back to sleep. It doesn't matter how good your sleep schedule is or how much caffeine you have cut out of your diet, it sometimes just happens. And, honestly there is nothing worse than lying in bed and staring at the ceiling simply because you just can't get yourself to fall back to sleep.

Now the worst part is when you start waking up every night and having a hard time going back to sleep. More than one night of this and your entire sleep schedule feels out of whack. Not to mention you spend several days dragging around being unproductive because you are so tired and have a hard time concentrating.

Rather than lying there night after night you need to take some kind of action to get yourself back to sleep. Luckily, there are several tips that you can follow to ensure you can get yourself back to sleep in record time.

- Don't think. If you wake up in the middle of the night, it is best to just lie still and stay in a relaxed position. No matter how tempting it might be don't start thinking about anything important. Don't even focus on the fact that you are having a hard time going back to sleep. All of this added stress is going to cause you to stay awake. Meditation or just mindfulness is a great way to prevent yourself from thinking.

- Relaxation techniques are a great way to help get yourself back to sleep. Sometimes if you try too hard to drift off back to sleep your body fights it. If you are lying there wide awake meditating, deep breathing, or visualization are great tools to use to help yourself relax. And while they are not a substitute for a good night's sleep, they can help rest and restore your body for the next day.

- Let's face it sometimes we lie there for what seems like forever with no luck. If you have been awake for more than 15 minutes try getting up out of bed and engaging your mind in something quiet and relaxing. Reading a book is one of the most relaxing things you can do in the middle of the night. No matter what you do though keep the lights down low, so as not to mess with your body's natural clock.

- One of the most common reasons why we wake up in the middle of the night is because we are worried about something; our subconscious mind tends to kick it out while we are sleeping. If this happens to you, don't stress over what you are worried about, as that will simply keep you up the rest of the night. Instead write down the reason you are worried about and revisit it in the morning. Same thing holds true if it is a brilliant idea that woke you up.

Dealing with a shift work schedule

Dealing with shift work, whether it is swing shift or grave yard shift, is one of the hardest things because your body is having to later its natural sleep schedule. While the most obvious choice would be to avoid these kinds of shifts, we all know that is not entirely possible, as not all of us have the luxury of working during the day.

If you find yourself having to do swing or grave yard shifts that doesn't mean you have to walk around in a daze while at work nor does it mean you have to live off of caffeinated drinks just to get you through the night. Here are some simple tips that you can put to use if you find yourself working these odd hours:

- Caffeine is something that most of us partake in as a way to wake ourselves up. If you must consume caffeine you want to do so early in your shift. Don't guzzle a 64 ounce soft drink 15 minutes before you head home, as that will cause sleep problems for sure.
- A steady work schedule is a great way to avoid sleep deprivation, which is quite common with these odd hour shifts. To help get a good night's rest either limit the number of crazy shifts you work in a row or try and avoid rotating shifts.
- Limit your commute as much as possible. If you have a super long commute that is going to cut into your sleeping time. Not to mention if you drive home during the day your body is going to slow down how much melatonin it is releasing, so you will become more alert and that makes it hard to sleep once you do get home.

- Change your sleep cycle. This is probably the single most important thing to do if you are working regular graveyard shifts. To start changing your sleep cycle you are going to need to expose yourself to bright lights as soon as you get up at night. You can also use daytime stimulating bulbs inside the workplace to help you stay awake and alert. Then when you are headed home use dark colored glasses to help reduce the amount of light you are exposed too, so your body starts producing melatonin.

Chapter Two:
Becoming A Morning Person After Being A Night Owl

Some people claim that they are naturally night owls, whether that is true or not has yet to be proven. However, I can tell you that going from late nights to early mornings is not going to be easy at all. Night owls love to stay up late, which requires sleeping late to ensure their body gets enough sleep. And, honestly, most night owls love and embrace that routine.

However, what happens when you have no choice but to become a morning person? How do you adopt a morning routine when you have become so used to a late afternoon/evening routine. Luckily, there are some useful tips that you can try out to help Make switching to a morning routine easier on both your mind and your body.

Create a pre-bed time routine

For former night owls often the hardest part of switching to a morning routine is getting into bed the night before at a decent time. They tend to lie awake tossing and turning for hours on end because their mind won't shut off. To help get yourself to bed earlier you need to create a pre-bedtime routine. When creating a pre-bedtime routine think about what kind of activities help you relax, such as a cup of tea or even a hot bath. Any kind of relaxing activities should be added to the routine, plus you will want to cut back on drinking too much alcohol at night, as well as caffeine after about dinner. Certain foods will also want to be avoided because of the havoc the cause your digestive system.

Think ahead

Before you go to bed sit down and think about what you have going on the next day. Setting an alarm or alert for a specific time each night to get ready for the next day is a great way to stay on top of getting it done. Once you have that figured out you can actually get the stuff ready that you will need first thing in the morning, such as laying out your clothes, preparing breakfast in the Crockpot, making your lunch, or putting everything you need in a specific place so you can quickly grab it on your way out the door in the morning. Getting everything ready the night before means you won't be scrambling trying to get it all done in the morning.

Organize your closet

This one might seem a little odd, but trust me when I say it will make your mornings go a lot smoother. Many of us simply hang stuff up helter skelter in our closets, which means we spend minutes rummaging through the clothes to find what we are looking for. However, if you take the time to organize your closet so that what you need during the week is right up front and ready to go you will save yourself several minutes each morning.

Follow your plan

When becoming a morning person, routine is key. Once you create your perfect morning routine, make sure that you follow it exactly each and every day. By following the same plan each day you are less likely to get distracted or surprised. You will always know what needs to be done and how long it takes to do it.

Limit distractions

One thing that can through a wrench into anybody's morning routine is distractions, whether it is the television or a computer. If part of your morning routine is to scan your email, do so, but avoid responding to anything until you have sat down and started working for the day. Not turning on the television is a great way to avoid becoming distracted. Becoming distracted tends to make you late or rushed in the morning, so you cut your routine a little short to help make up for lost time.

Follow your routine even on the weekends

Many people think that becoming a morning person is only something that needs to be done Monday through Friday. They figure the weekend all bets are off and its o.k. to stay up late and sleep in. However, that kind of defeats the purpose to create and following a morning plan because on Monday morning the weekend is going to end up catching up with you. To help make it easier to follow a morning routine you will want to stick with it even on the weekends. If you do want to "sleep in" do so by only 30 minutes or so.

Wake up shower

Not everybody ill agree with this one, but for those of you that enjoy aromatherapy you can put it to use to help you wake up and get energized in the morning. Whether you are taking a shower when you first get out of bed, after your morning workout, or even both you want to find scents for inside the shower that are sure to wake you up. You can purchase scented soaps, shampoos, and conditioners or you can purchase essential oils and add them to your favorite non-scented products or even diffuse them in the shower.

Chapter Three:
Getting Yourself Going In The Morning

Let's face it the single most important thing to creating or following a morning routine, is actually getting yourself going in the morning. You, yourself, know all too well just how hard it can be to get up out of bed during the mornings. Many of you probably find your bed to be one of the most comfortable places you have ever been. And the last thing you really want to do each morning is toss off the covers and hit the ground running.

Now no matter how warm and cozy you might be underneath those covers and no matter how cold and miserable it might be outside, you have to get up each morning and get moving. Now as unpleasant as this might sound, it really isn't all that bad. What makes it worse is procrastinating, so if you know a few tips and tricks that can help get you up and moving in the morning you are already ahead of the game.

Don't Hit Snooze

Now some people can wake up on time without an alarm clock. Some people can actually train themselves to follow a natural sleep cycle that allows them to wake up at the same time every day, while others will use what is called an internal alarm clock. However, for most of us we have to set an alarm to ensure we are getting up on time. If you are getting enough sleep each night though the alarm clock can be a just in case type thing. If you wake up before your alarm goes off, get up and get moving. If you rely heavily on your alarm clock the worst thing you can do is hit the dreaded snooze button.

If you are the type of person who loves to hit snooze, which honestly most people are, you need to take certain precautions with your alarm clock. To prevent hitting snooze repeatedly you want to place your alarm clock somewhere across the room, the further away the better. Having your alarm clock out of reach means you have to get up out of your bed to turn it off. The trick here is once you are up to stay up. Turn off the alarm and get ready to start your day instead of hitting snooze.

Leave your bedroom

Once you are up the key to staying up is to move away from your bedroom. Your bedroom is a place that your mind associates with sleep, so if you stay in there once you get up you are more likely to be tempted to go back to bed. If you get up, turn off your alarm and then immediately leave your bedroom you have a better chance at getting up and staying up.

Cold water

Some people say that getting into a nice, warm shower is a great way to wake up in the morning, but some people find the warm water to be a bit too relaxing. Once you are up and out of bed your best chance at helping yourself to wake up is to head straight out of your room and into the kitchen. In the kitchen pour yourself a nice, cold glass of water. You can pour on from the faucet or you can even keep a gallon of water inside the refrigerator, so it is really cold. The cold water will quench your thirst, plus will get your body moving as it will help wake up all of your internal organs.

Eat and drink the night before

Many people have a hard time getting up in the morning because they are groggy, their mind is in a fog and sometimes the best way to deal with that is going back to bed. For some people the reason they feel so off in the morning is because they have gone too long without eating. Now we are not saying to eat a huge meal full of fatty foods right before bed, but a late night snack is a good idea. When snacking at night make sure it is something small and easy to digest, such as cottage cheese or yogurt.

Now we just talked about drinking a glass of water first thing in the morning to help wake you up, but drinking water before bed is another good way to get up and moving in the morning. The reason for this is if you drink enough right before bed you will have to go to the bathroom in the morning, so when your alarm goes off you are less likely to hit snooze and crawl under the covers. Instead you are more likely to visit the bathroom before doing anything, which gives your body even more time to wake up. You will need to experiment with how much water you drink at night, as drinking too much will cause you to wake up in the middle of the night rather than first thing in the morning.

Open your blinds

Waking up in a dark room is not going to be very counterproductive if you want to get up and get moving in the morning. As the darkness makes it harder to wake up, you want nothing more than to crawl back into bed. This is really a struggle when it is still dark outside during the winter, so in those cases using bright lights as soon as you get out of bed is a great way to get moving in the morning.

If it is light outside when you normally wake up the easiest solution to let more light in, is to leave your blinds open at night while you are sleeping. Leaving them open allows the early morning sunlight to stream through and will shine down upon you. Once the sunlight starts streaming in you will find it harder to sleep. Plus the sunlight sends a message to your bodies that we are supposed to be up and moving.

Vitamins

In addition to eating a healthy breakfast to give your body the fuel it needs, you will also want to take a daily vitamin. Supplementing your diet with a good multivitamin ensures that your body is getting the vitamins and minerals it needs, which you will notice makes you feel more alert and energetic. If you are still feeling sluggish, pay close attention to how many B vitamins you are getting each day, you want to make sure you are getting the recommended dose. B vitamins are responsible for converting the food you eat into energy your body needs, not getting enough of these vitamins can make you feel like you are dragging.

Plan something for the morning

Whether it is an appointment or a date with a friend, having something planned will make it easier to get up and get moving. People find that when they are accountable for being somewhere at a certain time they are more motivated. Having that motivation is just enough to get you up and moving rather than crawling back under the covers.

Something else that will give you motivation to get up and get going in the morning is to plan something fun. If you have something fun to look forward to after getting up, you are more likely to have more energy and desire to get out of bed. Now planning something fun doesn't mean you have to leave the house, it can be just about anything that you enjoy doing, such as reading or playing video games.

No matter what motivating tips or tricks you might use to help get yourself up and moving in the morning it is best if you stick to some kind of a routine. Following a daily routine rather than just winging it every day allows your body to get into a natural rhythm, which will help you get a good night's rest, as well as have any easier time waking up in the morning.

Building Your Energy Each Morning

as you are probably already aware of building up your energy each morning is one of the biggest struggles to starting a morning routine. Majority of us, simply have no desire to get up and out of bed each morning. Some of us find it hard to get moving because we simply have no energy. To create energy several people revert to drinking coffee or something else with caffeine in it, as the caffeine is a stimulant and is sure to get your blood pumping. However, there are ways to build your energy in the morning without a jolt or two of caffeine.

As we have mentioned earlier in this chapter two of the best ways to get your energy levels up in the morning is to expose yourself to bright light as soon as you wake up and exercise. The bright light signals your body that it is time to be up and moving rather than sleeping, while the exercise is great at getting blood flowing and shaking off any excess sleepiness feelings.

Another great way to get your energy levels up in the morning is to follow what we like to call the ten minute rule. Once you get up in the morning you tend to sit on the edge of your bed and debate with yourself if you want to actually move from the bed. Most of the time you lose the debate and crawl under the covers, but that won't help when trying to establish a morning routine. Instead sit on the edge of your bed after your normal wake up time and stay there for 10 minutes. By resisting the urge to go back to bed for ten minutes chances are you won't have the urge any longer.

If you start the day using your mind actively rather than taking part in passive activities your energy levels will be higher. Focusing your mind early on in the morning has been proven to help you stay alert and focused throughout the remainder of the day. It also goes a long way towards shaking off any late downiness that may occur.

One of the worst habits we get into to help save time in the morning is to skip breakfast. However, this is not something that anybody really recommends, as breakfast is a very important meal. If you have to set your alarm so you get up a few minutes earlier so you can eat. Not eating can wreak havoc with your metabolism, but will also cause you to lose energy. Getting energy in the morning requires food, as it is the food that increases your blood sugar levels. And low levels result in lack of energy.

Finally, if you are really looking for a way to get up and moving in the early morning hours, crank up the volume. Whether you are listening to your favorite band or you are listening to the latest audio book, turning up the volume is a great way to get your blood pumping, especially if you find yourself dancing around the room as you get ready for the day.

Chapter Four:
Moving Around Wakes You Up

Getting up and going for a run in the morning before we've even had our first cup of coffee is not everyone's idea of a great morning exercise. In fact, you shouldn't be doing anything too strenuous until you've had time to stretch your muscles and release those amino acids from the various parts of your body to get you energized and feeling lithe. But first, let's get you some motivation to start doing morning exercises.

Here are nine interesting facts that will, hopefully, entice you to add exercise to your morning routine.

- Ninety percent of those who exercise in the morning exercise consistently.

- Those who exercise in the morning jumpstart their metabolism and sometimes it stays elevated for twenty-four hours.

- You'll feel more energized for the day and be able to think quicker than someone who hasn't exercised in the morning.

- Exercising in the morning will put you into a healthy mindset and you won't find yourself overeating or eating unhealthy foods at lunch and dinner.

- By exercising in the morning, you will actually regulate your circadian and endocrine rhythms and this will lead you to getting a better night's sleep and waking up more refreshed in the morning.

o When your endocrine and circadian rhythms actually have a rhythm, it's much easier to wake up when your alarm clocks goes off in the morning.

o You feel more alert in the morning when you wake up because your endocrine system is awake before you are.

- Many find that it's a good time to think about the rest of their day and plan ahead.

- People who exercise in the morning increase their mental acuity, and it can last anywhere from four to ten hours after exercise.

- Exercising in the morning is the best for your schedule because it ensures that nothing else will take precedence over it.

- People who exercise on a regular basis have a high quality of sleep and actually require less sleep every night.

Now that you have some incentive, which exercises are best to do in the morning if you're just beginning to exercise? And which exercise burn more calories and leave you feeling more alert? Well, here's a chart to let you know how many calories you can burn if you're interested in losing weight, and then I'll give you an example exercise routine that involves stretching, minor cardio, and some weight lifting if you're feeling particularly adventurous.

Exercise Type	Calories Burned	Amount of Time
Running/Jogging (5 MPH)	295	30 Minutes
Bicycling (10 MPH)	195	30 Minutes
Swimming	255	30 Minutes
Aerobics	240	30 Minutes
Basketball	220	30 Minutes
Walking (3.5 MPH)	140	30 Minutes
Weight Training	110	30 Minutes
Stretching	90	30 Minutes
Biking	145	30 Minutes
Dancing	165	30 Minutes

So now that you know how many calories you're burning, let's take a look at a beginner's routine, and then we'll add in some more strenuous exercises for those who already exercise during the day but want to add a routine to their morning schedule.

For Beginners

For those who are looking for exercises that will help them wake up and get their blood flowing, but won't make them feel as if they've run a marathon, these are some excellent exercise choices.

Back Stretch

This is actually a yoga exercise that will help you strengthen your back as well as get your digestive system moving. Simply lie on your back on the floor or a yoga mat and hug both your knees to your chest. Then raise your head and shoulders off the floor and hold this position for fifteen seconds, breathing deeply by raising your abdomen up and down rather than using your chest. Then release slowly and repeat this exercise ten times with ten second breaks in between, and do four repetitions.

Cat-Cow Position

It sounds a bit odd, but the cat-cow movement will help strengthen your core, as well as stretch out your back muscles and your abdominal muscles. Start by lying down on your stomach and bring yourself up into a kneeling position with your hands on the floor in front of you. Then inhale and tuck your tailbone as you round your back and look toward your belly button. Then exhale and drop your belly as you arch your lower back and look up.

Do this ten times and repeat the sets of ten four times.

Shoulder Stretch

This is an excellent way to get yourself motivated just as you get out of bed, or a good way to cool down after a long workout. Simply reach your right hand back over your should and reach your left hand back behind you. Then clasp your hands together and hold this position for ten to fifteen seconds. Then switch to your left hand over your shoulder and your right hand behind your back and hold again. Repeat this four times.

Intermediate Positions

If you're looking to build some muscle and lose a little weight, as well as tone your body, then these exercises should help. Keep in mind that doing a few stretches before you begin these is a good idea as they can be strenuous when you first start out.

Prisoner Squat

To perform the prisoner squat, stand with your feet shoulder width apart and be sure that your posture is correct. Then put your hands behind your head as if you're being arrested, and lower your body with your hips back and bend your knees. Go down as far as you can. Pause for a few seconds, and then slowly push back up to the starting position. Do this four times with one minute breaks in between and ten repetitions.

The High Kneed Walk

Stand with your feet shoulder width apart and make sure your back is straight. Then, without changing how you're standing, raise your left knee as high as possible and step forward. Do not round your lower back. Repeat with your right leg and do this for thirty seconds.

The Mount Climber

Get on your hands and knees and then assume the pushup position with your arms straight. Lift your right leg off the floor and bring it as close to your chest as you can. Then touch the floor with your right foot. Go back to the starting position and repeat with your left leg. Then alternate back and forth for thirty seconds. Do ten repetitions.

Experienced

Once you've moved past working out with just your own body weight, you've moved into the experienced category. Now, in order to get yourself into shape, you must use hands weights or dumbbells. Try starting out with just one pound dumbbells and moving up incrementally as you become comfortable.

The Dumbbell Squat

This is exactly like the intermediate squat except you're adding weights. Hold the weights in your hands and assume the position with your feet placed shoulder width apart and tighten your abdominal muscles as you stand straight. Then lower your body as far as you can and pause. Rise back up slowly and repeat ten times.

The Row

This is definitely one that can become difficult if you're a beginner, so be aware of how far to push your body and don't go too crazy with this one. Hold your dumbbells in your hands and stand up straight. Then lower yourself as if you're sitting in a chair and hold that position. Your arms should be loose and your palms should be facing behind you. Then bring the dumbbells up to the side of your torso and pause. Slowly lower them back. Repeat this ten times.

Chapter Five:
Affirmations during Hygienic Routine

After waking up and doing your exercises, taking a shower is probably in order. But did you know that you can kill two birds with one stone? While you're taking a relaxing shower, why not repeat some of your daily affirmations to yourself? Let's take a look at why so many people are starting to repeat affirmations and how you can come up with a few on your own.

What is an affirmation, and why should I use them?

Affirmations are a series of words that usually form a sentence saying something about yourself or something you want to happen, and they're aimed at affecting your conscious and your subconscious mind. At this point, you might be asking if this is brainwashing yourself. In fact, it's a little like that, except these are positive things that will eventually become a reality for you because everything you do throughout the day is aiming at making those affirmations come true.

What do they do?

Affirmations should be motivating in order to get you to do the tasks you need to accomplish in order to complete your goal. Therefore, an affirmation should be aimed at keeping you on track. If you're using them properly, they will activate the subconscious mind and the powers that are within your mind lying dormant.

An affirmation will ultimately change the way you think, the way you behave, and bring you into contact with new people and new goals. They should make you feel positive and energized when you're finished saying them.

When should I say them and how many times?

You can say them at any time during the day, but the best times to say them are before you go to bed and during your morning routine. You can choose to say them during your hygiene routine or you can choose to say them as you're visualizing or meditating, or even when you first wake up in order to get yourself motivated to get out of bed. You may even choose to repeat them as many times as you wish throughout the day.

Before you begin, though, you should ask whether or not you actually want what you're going to ask for. If there's any doubt that you want what you're asking for, you will stand in the way of yourself. Therefore, be sure you want that job promotion before you begin.

Use love, faith, feeling, and interest when you are affirming. Talk as if you have already fulfilled the affirmation rather than saying that it *will* happen. By doing this, you are accelerating the fulfillment of the affirmation.

What are some examples of affirmations?

You can choose to use these affirmations specifically if they really speak to you, but really you ought to change them to suit your needs. By making them personal, you are making them resonate more with your subconscious.

- For Success

    o I can achieve success because it is simple and easy.

    o Success is always seeking me.

- I can feel success flowing into my life.

- I am achieving my goals.

- Every time I inhale, I am filling with prosperity, and every time I exhale, I am ridding myself of failure.

- Happiness

  - Happiness is manifesting in my life right now.

  - I deserve to be happy and will be happy.

  - Happiness is seeking me.

  - I am breathing in happiness and breathing out depression.

  - I am happy right now.

- Health

  - I am functioning perfectly and all my systems are happy.

  - Healing energy is filling me right now.

  - I can feel the universe filling me with healing energy.

  - Each cell of my body is filled with healing energy and singing with happiness.

  - My health is improving day by day.

- Money

  - Money is flowing into my life freely.

  - I am obtaining more and more money daily.

  - I am a money magnet.

  - The universe is sending more money my way daily.

  - I am earning a lot of money.

- Self-Confidence

  - I am beautiful.

  - I am worthy of being loved.

  - Many people love me.

  - The universe is sending a lot of love my way.

  - I am important.

Notice how each of these affirmations focuses on the person as an individual and is specific about their concerns. Repeat these to yourself out loud as you're doing your hair or makeup in the mirror, or do them mentally as you're brushing your teeth. You'll feel clean inside and out when you're doing your affirmations as you're doing your daily hygiene routine.

Chapter Six:
Eating a Healthy Breakfast

You've heard the saying that breakfast is the most important meal of the day, but do you know why? Most of us took it upon good faith because our mothers told us to eat breakfast because it would help us grow up strong and healthy, and they weren't wrong. Breakfast is the most important meal of the day because it is the meal that breaks your fast from food overnight, which brings your body out of ketosis. Ketosis is the state in which our bodies burn fat rather than calories we're eating, and what better way to break that fast than to put something really healthy into our systems?

Eating a healthy breakfast is linked to weight control, better performance throughout the day, strength and endurance during physical activities, and lower cholesterol levels. That translates to a healthier, better you. So don't skip the morning meal and make it a good one!

Here are some tips on how to make your breakfasts healthier.

Add Protein

Did you know that protein is an essential building block of the body's cells? It's also the best food to help blunt hunger because ultimately our bodies are craving protein and not much else. When we eat enough protein, our minds immediately tell our bodies we're no longer hungry.

The traditional breakfast of eggs is actually one of the best things you can eat. Those commercials and the food companies are not lying to you, for once. They're telling the truth when eggs are packed full of vitamins and protein. If that's not convincing enough, one study conducted by

Pennington Biomedical Research Center had two groups, overweight women who ate bagels for breakfast and overweight women who ate eggs for breakfast. The calories between the eggs and the bagel were actually the same amount, yet the women who ate eggs lost sixty-five percent more weight.

In addition to being great for weight loss, eggs actually make you feel fuller quicker and longer. Therefore, you spend less time agonizing what you're going to be eating for lunch and more time working on that project you know you have to get done. So if you don't have any serious heart problems or cholesterol issues eat two eggs for breakfast and even add a slice of bacon.

The Truth about Cereal

I'm not talking about Captain Crunch or Cocoa Puffs. They're okay as a snack occasionally, but you should really be eating some healthy, whole grain cereals, and they should have no added sugar, too. A Harvard study of over 17,000 men determined that men who ate breakfast cereal frequently weighed less than those who didn't eat breakfast cereal.

As long as it's a healthy cereal and a reasonable amount, breakfast cereal will actually make you feel full and energized throughout the morning.

So What about Other Foods?

I'm glad you asked. There are so many different foods you can eat for breakfast that are healthful and beneficial to your body! This is just a short list of common foods that you can try out for breakfast. Find a few favorites and get started having a healthy, energizing breakfast tomorrow morning.

- Some whole-wheat toast with a vegetable omelet.

- A homemade breakfast sandwich consisting of a whole-wheat English muffin, cheese, a scrambled egg, and a slice of tomato or maybe ham.

- A smoothie with yogurt and fruit.

- A whole-grain bagel with cream cheese and a slice of smoked salmon.

- Some whole-grain cereal with fruit and milk.

- A glass of orange juice and some oatmeal with raisins and nuts.

- Some fruit in low-fat yogurt.

- A breakfast bar.

- A banana and a hard-boiled egg.

- Half a grapefruit.

- A slice of whole-wheat bread with almond butter.

- A cup of blueberries.

Pretty much any type of fruit is healthy to eat for breakfast, and something that has protein such as yogurt, peanut butter, almond butter, Nutella, any meat or eggs. The list is almost endless to what you can eat for breakfast every morning.

A quick note; some people prefer to eat a light breakfast before they start working out. There aren't any benefits to eating breakfast before or directly after a workout, so it's really a personal preference. However, your body is going to need protein in order to replenish the muscles you just broke down, so keep that in mind the next time you're heading for a donut. Those aches in your arms and legs will go away much quicker with an egg than a pastry.

Chapter Seven:
Visualization before Starting the Day and Meditation for Stress Relief

Meditation and visualization are not interchangeable. They are two vague concepts that have to be narrowed down to your specific values and basically how your mind works on a subconscious level. For example, one person might need movement during meditation while another might need absolute stillness. In this chapter, I'm going to touch on some basic visualization and meditation techniques, but don't be afraid to look outside of this source for other types in order to find one that works best for you.

First, let's talk about what meditation is and why you should be doing it. Meditation is basically a state of deep concentration where your mind is being given one point of focus rather than bouncing around from one topic to the next. A lot of people give up on this practice because they are constantly thinking about other things as they're meditating, but it takes practice and concentration on the body rather than the mind to succeed. But once you do, you'll wonder why it took you so long to try this in the first place!

Now, let's discuss visualization. Visualization is actually a form of meditation, but you're focusing on an image. There are two different forms, visual or kinesthetic. A kinesthetic visualization is creating the experience of actually doing something within your mind. You will *feel* yourself going through that action using all five of your senses. This might be an image of you obtaining a job promotion or just something as simple as having a wonderful day. The other type of visualization, visual, is picturing a sequence of events or another person, but you're not really feeling it. The best type of visualization is both visual and kinesthetic.

There are forms of meditation that combine with visualization, but there are meditation techniques that do not involve visualization at all. In fact, they shy away from picturing any type of image because this is considered a thought. So let's discuss both techniques separately in great detail so that you fully understand what you are doing.

Visualization

Visualization is used to either relieve stress or bring about subconscious actions that will get you to where you want to go. For example, visualization that is for relaxation might include a picture of a calming place or a place that feels safe for you, such as a calming landscape or a deserted beach. Visualization can be used for healing, such as visualizing that the heart is working calmly and healthily. It can be used for performing an action perfectly such as scoring a goal in a soccer game. It can be used for mapping out what you're going to do and say during a business meeting in order to obtain a client or impress the boss.

When you're using visualization in meditation, your mind is concentrating as your physical body is relaxing. So in order to practice it, you should be sitting down in a comfortable position or even lying down, and you should be picturing and feeling what you're going to do that day. Leave all negative aspects out of your visual in order to bring about positives during the day.

You can also do this at night before you go to bed. It's an excellent technique to use when you're visualizing all the positive things you did that day and all the positive things you're going to do in the morning. While you're doing this, you should be breathing in an out evenly in order to remain in a calm, relaxed state.

Here's a step by step guide to get you started.

- Clear your mind and concentrate on your breathing.

- Create or imagine your visual image or feeling before you start this exercise, and then bring it up and relive it repeatedly as you're breathing.

- As you inhale, imagine your body is expanding with potential and as you exhale your positive thoughts are being expelled into the world. They're planting their seeds in order for you to have a successful day.

Meditation

Meditation, also known as mindfulness, is a mental practice that involves concentration and mantras or focusing on the breaths. It's particularly helpful for those who are under a lot of stress or can't seem to calm their minds enough to do their daily routine. Some choose to practice meditation as soon as they get out of bed while others choose to practice this technique just before they go off to work to start the day.

Here are some things to remember as you're meditating.

- Don't force it. Once you've obtained concentration, don't judge the thoughts or observations within your mind as either good or bad. Just let them flow by with a brief acknowledgment.

- Pay attention to what's happening inside your mind. You will notice things happening outside of your person such as sounds, sights, and feelings but don't allow those to distract you. Instead, focus on what's happening within your mind.

- Keep it up. Sometimes it takes a little while for your mind to adjust to this process. It might seem alien to you at first and frustrating, but don't give up. Give it at least thirty days in order to see if it's something that you can build into a habit.

- Redirect your thoughts. Sometimes they might wander to planning, daydreaming or even criticism of what you're doing, but redirect your mind to the present and what you should be visualizing.

Now with those thoughts in mind, let's take a look at some common mindfulness meditation techniques that you can start using in the morning.

Basic Meditation

This is something that all beginners should start with as it's very simple and uses a focal point that is easy to concentrate on.

1. Find a comfortable position in a chair or sit cross-legged on the floor.

2. Place your right hand on your abdomen and your left hand on your chest. Now breathe through your nostrils and count to four as you're doing so. You should be using your abdomen to breathe in and your chest should not be moving much. Then hold that breath for seven seconds. Now exhale through your mouth for eight seconds.

3. Once you've fully concentrated on your breathing, you can let some of the outside inside. Listen to the sounds, sensations, and the ideas within you.

4. Remember not to judge any thoughts that come into your mind. Simply acknowledge them and allow them to pass.

5. If you find your mind is skipping from one topic to another, focus on your breathing again and start over.

Informal Meditation

Sometimes you need to start off with an introductory period before you start going directly into mindfulness meditation. It's reasonable to start off with only twenty minutes in the morning rather than going the entire forty-five minute length most professionals or experienced meditators do. It takes about twenty minutes for the mind to begin to calm; therefore, you should experience a calming feeling just before you're finished. Try some of these techniques to begin with if you're not comfortable with the previously mentioned method.

- Start by trying to practice while you're eating, showering, walking, or playing with your children.

- Concentrate on the sensations in your body and what you're currently sensing with all five senses.

- Breathe in through your nose and let your abdomen expand fully.

- Then breathe out through your mouth.

- Note how you feel as you inhale and exhale.

- Keep doing the task you were doing before but do it with full deliberation.

- Engage each sense (sight, sound, touch, taste, and smell) so that you can recall them later.

Chapter Eight:
Tips for Creating the Perfect Morning Routine

If you are having a hard time getting going in the morning or if you wake up every morning feeling overwhelmed, you night want to seriously consider adopting some kind of morning routine. One of the things that you might not realize is that how you start your morning off, generally reflects how you are going to spend the rest of your day. So, if you start off rushing around trying to get things done in some kind of panicked state, you are going to find yourself rushing around the rest of the day.

Creating a morning routine is the best way to get a handle on your mornings, as well as the rest of your day. Now for those of you who were not raised following any specific routines, the thought of trying to create a morning routine can be a bit overwhelming. But, trust me, it is totally worth doing and it will give you back control of your day.

One of the hardest parts of creating a morning routine is coming up with something that works for you. However, once you do come up with something that works for you, you will be happier with your life. Creating the perfect morning routine gives you control over your life; it gives you the opportunity to do more of the things you love because you know have the time to do it. Now creating the perfect routine is not going to happen overnight. To make your routine a habit you are going to need to follow it every single day, consistency is key with routines.

Here are some useful tips that you can follow to create the perfect morning routine for you.

Get up early

One of the best things you can do to help create a perfect routine for you is to get yourself up before everybody else in your house. Getting up before everybody means you are not rushing around trying to get everything done from the moment your feet hit the floor. You are giving yourself some time to yourself. This is helpful as it allows you to wake up and get ready at your own pace without having to worry about everything else.

Morning cup of coffee

Now this one isn't going to apply to everybody, but for those of you that enjoy having a morning cup of coffee doing so during your alone time is the perfect way to help get going. However, don't just limit yourself to a cup of coffee; you also want to hydrate yourself with a glass of water. After sleeping all night, water is a great way to wake up your body, as your organs need water to function properly. If you prefer something else in the morning, such as soda or even a glass of juice, it is still helpful to add a glass of water to the routine.

Connect with yourself

As we mentioned earlier in this eBook meditation is a great way to get in touch with your inner self in the morning, but it is not the only way. It's not as important as to how you do it, but rather that you take the time to connect with yourself each and every day. Other ideas of being able to connect with yourself include taking a morning walk, stretching, or even yoga. Getting connected with yourself is all about making yourself feel good and ready to take on your day.

Plan your day

Knowing what you have to accomplish during the day makes it easier to get everything done. Not to mention planning your day when you get up allows for everything to flow smoothly. Now how you plan your day is going to depend on what kind of day you have to plan. One of the most effective ways to plan out a day is to create a to do list first thing in the morning. What is important here isn't how you do it, but that you account for everything that needs to get done.

Down time

When you plan out your day chances are you only think of what needs to get done. When creating your list of stuff that needs to get done, it is all too easy to overlook giving yourself some much needed down time. As you plan out your day make sure you set aside a small block of time to do something that you enjoy, something that isn't related to responsibility, such as painting or reading a book.

When creating a morning routine you are going to have to practice it every day, as like we mentioned earlier, consistency is key in creating a routine. The tips that we mentioned above are useful in creating the perfect morning routine, but they are not set in stone. You can add to this list or take away from it to create something that works for you.

Chapter Nine:
Creating a Family Friendly Morning Routine

Having a family is a lot of hard work, whether you are a stay at home parent or a working parent, getting things ready to go in the morning can be rather difficult. Many parents wake up and find themselves having to rush about to get everything done and even then they find themselves constantly running behind or stressed out. If you as a parent find yourself overwhelmed each morning trying to get everything situated its time to think about creating a morning routine for both you and your family.

By taking the time to create a morning routine for your family you are creating a secure environment for your family. A secure environment allows everybody to know what their roles and responsibilities are in the household, so they know what to expect each day. Morning routines are the best way to give you and your family calm and ordered life.

Now when you are getting ready to create a morning routine for your family you want to keep three things in mind: specific tasks, specific order, and consistency. Specific tasks need to be kept in mind because you need to know what needs to be done and how long it takes to do them. The specific order refers to how you are going to go about doing your specific tasks. When creating the order it makes sense to do so based on priority or a logical sequence. And consistency is the single most important thing to keep in mind because without it you will never be able to successfully adopt a morning routine for your family.

Many people often avoid creating a morning routine because they simply have no idea where to start. If that is the case with you, don't run from it, simply embrace your fear and move forward. Creating a morning routine isn't hard, if you break it down into smaller sections. Think about what has to be done and who is going to do it.

If you are seriously struggling to come up with a morning routine for your family to follow, here are a few general ideas that can help you get started.

- **Waking Up** – Don't just jump up out of bed and hit the ground running, as that can lead to a chaotic day. Instead set aside 10 to 15 minutes to allow yourself to wake up, even if it means setting the alarm clock 15 minutes early. Prepping your coffee the night before so it is ready when you wake up in the morning is a great way to get the day started.

- **Go over your schedule** – After you have woke up mentally go over all of the things that you need to get done during the day. It even helps creating a to do list the night before, so you can read it over first thing in the morning.

- **Make your bed** – For many people this is a no brainer, but you might be surprised at how many people simply neglect to make their beds each morning. Many of you have the theory you are going to mess it up again that night, so why bother making it in the morning. The reason behind making your bed in the morning is it makes the room look less cluttered, which gives you peace of mind.

- **Get kids ready for school** – This is one of the most time consuming tasks during the day, how long it takes will depend on how many kids you have, as well as their ages. In some cases you can assign different tasks to older children to help make the process easier. But getting ready for school means waking kids up, feeding them breakfast, brush their teeth, and get all of the bags ready.

- **Breakfast** – If you are a stay at home parent this can be done after getting the kids off to school or it can be done before, just depends on what works out best for your schedule. Just remember part of making breakfast is also cleaning up afterwards. Cleaning the kitchen after each meal makes it look less cluttered; this is actually less stressful, as its one less thing for you to worry about doing during the day. Plus coming home to a clean kitchen after a long day at work is actually quite relaxing.

- **Prepare for dinner** – Again where you fit this in your schedule will depend on how you set up your schedule. But preparing for dinner involves making sure everything is pulled out of the freezer and ready to go, as well as making sure you have everything you need or if you need to plan a trip to the grocery store. Meal planning makes dinner prep a lot easier, as you have a ready to go menu to easily refer too.

- **Dishes** – Emptying the dishwasher and dish drainer first thing in the morning allows you to easily keep up on dishes throughout the day. Plus it frees up some time faster dinner as there aren't nearly as many dishes to do.

When creating your morning routine for your family you can base it off this list or you can add to it. What kind of morning routine you create will depend on what you need to get done in the morning. The important thing to remember is that once you have completed your morning routine, you need to move on with your day, whatever it is that you have planned.

Chapter Ten:
Upgrading Your Morning Routine

Creating a basic morning routine that works for you and your family is not that hard. However, even the best of us find that our morning routines don't always work. Even after weeks of consistently following our morning routines we still find ourselves rushing about, our days seem to be even more stressful, if that is even possible. So, what do you do when you determine that your morning routine just isn't working for you? Do you continue to just follow it and hope everything works itself out? No, you don't. If your morning routine is no longer working you need to take matters into your own hand. It's time to upgrade your morning routine.

So, what does upgrading your morning routine entail, you ask? Well the answer is relatively simple. To upgrade your morning routine you are going to need to rethink your current morning routine. You want to look at what you are doing and seeing what needs to be fixed or if you can substitute something else for what you are currently doing.

Here are a few upgrades to consider for your new morning routine.

Track your current routine

If you are still finding yourself rushed and hurried each morning you need to seriously sit down and figure out what is going on. The best way to do this is to really track all of your morning tasks to see what is taking up so much of your time. Once you get handle on what is taking up so much time you can revise your routine so you are no longer rushed. Sometimes it means fewer distractions, while sometimes you might not be getting up early enough. The better you know what needs to be done and how long it takes, the easier it will be to create a routine to follow that works.

Create a routine for your kids

Even if you have your morning routine perfectly planned out, your kids can always throw a wrench into it. Kids are famous for constantly taking their time to get things done or even using the excuse of one more minute. Having to wait on kids or get kids moving causes routines to go out the window, unless you put your kids on a routine as well. If they are having a hard time getting ready in the morning because of watching cartoons, simply turn off the television. Plus creating a routine for them to follow, even if it takes days to get everything working right, will make it less stressful for both you and your kids.

Thinking

As you are probably already aware of the early morning hours are often the quietest of the day, especially if you get up before everybody in your home. Reserve these quiet hours for thinking through things. Use this time to silently work through any problems that you might be having, whether at work or at home. You can also work on any challenges that you are currently facing, as the quiet is a great time to come up with some winning solutions.

Prioritize

One thing that you can do will sitting in the quiet of the morning is to learn how to prioritize your tasks. Many people start their day off by looking over their email, but the truth is there are often more pressing things that need to be done. What you need to do is work on the most important thing on your list first thing each morning. Emails that came through at the end of the day are often not as pressing as some of your other tasks. Doing your most important task before you even check your email will make you feel like you have had a productive morning.

Use caffeine wisely

Many people who use caffeine to jump start their mornings drink way too much at once, so it is not nearly as effective. Rather than going for that extra large cup of coffee in the mornings, which will simply give you the shakes, try drinking a few smaller cups of coffee spaced throughout the morning. Or switching to diet soda or tea gives you the smaller doses. Or if you are feeling adventurous you can start your day off without any kind of caffeine.

Prep the night before

No matter how much we micromanage our mornings sometimes they are just hectic because we have so much going on. To take the load off in the mornings it is often times helpful to prep as much stuff the night before as possible. You can often throw a breakfast dish into the Crockpot to cook overnight; you can get the coffee maker ready so your cup is already brewed when you wake up. You can even create a to do list the night before of what needs to be done the next day, so you can review it first thing in the morning. It doesn't matter what you prep or how much you prep the night before, all that matters is you do it to take some of the stress off the mornings.

Know Your Peak Times

One of the best ways to upgrade your morning routine is to start your day off when you know you are going to have the most energy. Knowing your peak performances times allows you to create and schedule things based on when they are most likely to get done. For some of us this is not possible, as we can't rearrange our work hours, but you can prioritize your work stuff based on your energy levels during your scheduled work day.

Chapter Eleven:
A Simple Morning Routine That Everyone Can Follow

Now we have spent this entire book talking about how important it is to create a morning routine. We have also mentioned a few different things that you can include in a morning routine, as well as tips on how to upgrade your morning routine if the first one you created isn't working for you. However, what we haven't really covered is what an actual morning routine looks like.

One of the greatest things about a morning routine is that they do not have to be complicated. In fact, the more complicated you make your morning routine the harder it is going to be to follow it. When creating a morning routine you want something that is going to be easy to implement, as that will increase the chances of you sticking with it even on the weekends when you are not as rushed. And as we all know consistency is key to creating a morning routine that actually works.

So rather than spend hours agonizing over creating the perfect morning routine, here is a simple morning routine that everybody can follow.

Stretch

This is something that most adults simply don't do when they first wake up, as they are often in the mindset of how much stuff they have to get done. Instead of bouncing out of bed and hitting the ground running, take a few minutes to allow yourself to wake up, which includes stretching and yawning as you lie in bed.

Stay away from the phone

With how much technology has advanced over the years more and more people are using their phones as an alarm clock. Instead of using your phone you can easily get into the habit of using an older styled alarm clock and just setting your phone for back up. However, no matter what type of alarm you have set you need to stay away from your phone in the mornings. All too often we grab our phone and start scrolling through all of the notifications we see on our lock screens, which then leads off to check on various apps. This is a practice that wastes several minutes, if not half an hour in a single sitting. Instead of focusing on the phone, which leads you to check your email, first thing in the morning, satisfy yourself with your thoughts. You will also find that it helps lower your stress level in the morning, which makes mornings go even better.

Water

Most of us find ourselves going for that early morning cup of coffee or even a cold soda to get our day started, after all a jolt of caffeine is a great way to open up your eyes and get the blood flowing. However, that is not the best choice for your first drink of the morning, especially after going at least 8 hours without drinking anything. Instead of caffeine drink at least an 8 ounce glass of water as soon as you wake up. It is amazing how that one simple drink will make you feel, both physically and mentally.

High protein snack/meal

Now throughout this eBook we have mentioned how important it is to have a good, healthy breakfast. Your body has gone at least 8 hours, preferably more since you don't want to eat very late at night, so it is seriously lacking in terms of fuel. To start your morning off right your body needs fuel, but you want to make sure you choose the right kind of foods. If you aren't much of a breakfast eater, either because you don't like to cook early in the morning or you just aren't that hungry, the worst thing you can do is skip breakfast or grab a snack that is too sugary or full of carbs. Instead of a bagel or even a waffle, grab something that is high in protein. Carbs and sugary foods might fill you up in the beginning, but after about an hour your body will have burned off the carbs and sugar and you will feel hungry again. Not to mention sugary foods often lead to a sugar crash. Protein shakes are a great choice for a meal replacement, as they fill you up and leave you feeling full until around lunch time.

Head outdoors

Many of us love to hit the snooze button in the morning. We have falsely allowed ourselves to believe that by hitting snooze we are actually getting a few extra minutes of sleep, in most cases snooze last for 15 minutes. But, like I said, we falsely believe we are getting more sleep. When your alarm first goes off you are yanked out of REM sleep, which is the restful sleep your body needs to rejuvenate itself. When you hit snooze your body simply doesn't have enough time to enter back into that deep sleep, so you are simply resting rather than sleeping. So what can you do instead of hitting snooze? Easy get up and head outside for a 15 minute walk. The best part about taking a quick walk is all you have to do is get dressed, no extra effort is involved. Walking outside in the fresh air will not only wake you up, it will also get your blood pumping so you are ready to tackle the rest of your day. As a side note, the 15 minute power walk is also a great way to kick start your metabolism, which helps if you are trying to lose weight.

Now this is just a sample of what a morning routine can look like, but it is an easy one to get stated with. With this morning routine you can add to it or you can substitute one thing for another. The important thing is to create something that you will want to follow each morning, something that will make you feel like you are getting your day started with less stress. As we mentioned before a great way to reduce your stress each morning is to prepare for the morning the night before, laying out clothes, reviewing your calendar, and even planning your day. The more you get done the night before, the less you have to do the next morning.

If you do decide to create your own morning routine something to keep in mind is that when creating one you are basically just substituting something productive for something unproductive. And for all of you people out there who have resisted creating and following a morning routine because you thought it would require a lot of work, this example just how little time and effort are actually involved.

Conclusion

Thank you for reading The Morning Ritual! Hopefully, you've learned how to get your morning started off right by implementing a nightly routine, waking up on time at the same time every morning, starting to exercise, using affirmations, eating healthy, and practicing meditation. Let's take a look at an example routine in order to get you started on the right path.

1. Wake up at 6AM.

2. Stretch for fifteen minutes.

3. Workout for thirty minutes.

4. Say ten affirmations while showering.

5. Eating breakfast and repeat five more affirmations.

6. Meditate for half an hour.

7. Visualize my day for fifteen minutes before heading off to work.

You can change around the routine to fit your needs and your preferences, but be sure to include the exercise, a healthy breakfast, meditation, and affirmations in order to get your day started off right. Remember that a morning routine is not just to get you out the door on time; it's about making you feel positive, healthy, and ready for the rest of your day. And don't forget to create a nighttime ritual in order to wake up feeling refreshed in the morning already.

If you liked this book, please take the time to log onto the retailer you bought it from and leave a positive review!

Thank you and have a good morning!

3 Chapters of:

Pilates

Get the Body You Always Wanted, Right Now

Chapter 1:
The need for body trimming

None of us can deny the pressures on our souls because of these fast moving life patterns. All day long we move from one place to another, for working deadlines, household chores and special agreements. This has made the human life more liable towards robotic routines. Every rising sun is having some different and variant challenge. Many people owe this extensive development and progress of mankind in the field of technology and research. As more and more aspects are being conquered, the challenges for humans are also becoming gigantic. So in this tiresome war of survival, the human beings have nearly forgotten their existence and the need for taking care of one's self.

Apart from various needs like the physiological and the need for accomplishment, there have are innumerable reasons which can be listed for making the human posture fit and trim.

> **The tiresome routines**

As discussed in the introductory notes, human life is no less than a challenge. In this venture of financial struggle many of us have become ignorant for their individualistic needs. Spending hours and hours sitting on our workstations, in a need to earn more and to get prominent position in one's corporate and social circle, we have left our self far away. Other than physical fatigue, all this tiresome challenge has posed a number of questions for the quality of life. While planning our lives, we should account for a balanced approach, an approach which can aid us in meeting the both ends. One major thing which needs to be accounted for is the dependency of this entire struggle on human health. So while on our way to challenging work life, we should also keep an eye on the need for keeping our body slim and trim.

➤ The decreased immunity level

As all pictures having two side of analysis, the technology outburst has also given birth to a number of major aftermaths pertaining to human life. All these points are interconnected. The demanding routine of work has made individuals less concerned towards their body needs. As a result the dependency over processed and easy to eat food has increased to a horrible level. All the artificial food and processed diet patterns has made the human body internally weak, so much so that the munity level against the infections and bacterial attacks has reduced to an alarming level.

➤ Reliance on technology big cut to physical activity

Yet another aftermath of this technology dependent human world has been observed in the shape of reduced physical activity. We have become surrounded by machines, robots and digital assistants. Form mobile phone to large space rockets all the inventions of technology has drastically altered the human routine. The increased dependency on machines has led to extremely low levels of physical activities. So the human body has become addict of no physical output. All work is done through workstations, with just a few clicks. From shopping to planning everything is mechanized form ordering to online delivery. All this has put human far from physical activity and more inclined towards obesity and health issues.

➤ Overweight denotes social humiliation

Connecting all these major points ne major consequence is the increased trend of obesity and being overweight. The story does not end here. In fact it is the commencement of a new quandary. Because of having a detracted body, many of us have to encounter blunt remarks and humiliating statements. It is a severe trauma for the individual suffering from it, as he has a sturdy routine, and is not equipped to spend any of his time for his body trimming. The situation become even worse if re affected individual is a female. Female being highly possessive about body shape and beauty become extremely fatigued about this matter, the social mortification faced by being overweight leads towards the mental and emotional disturbances. So the need for body trimming has heightened greatly.

Chapter 2:
The Emergence of Pilates- Setting Miraculous Standards for Human World

Pilates is a term used for an exclusive classification of strengthening, stabilizing and stretching exercises, introduced about ninety years ago by Joseph H. Pilates, who was basically a German born. He was a physical culturist. The history of his upbringing strongly connotes his interest in the field of physical arts, as his mother was a naturopath and his father worked for long as a gymnast. His father won a number if pries and distinction in this filed. Being brought up in such an environment, Pilates naturally had the tendency to get interested in physical arts and exercises. He learned and practiced varying categories of exercise including yoga, both Eastern trends as well as the Western forms of exercise.

Earlier in his youth, he was skillful in a number of physical training regimes, which were practiced at that time in Germany. All this summed up for his inspiration for developing the idea of Pilates. These were the time traced back to late ninetieth century when the physical culture was taking a turn and the use of exercises as a preventive as well as a curative technique, was gaining momentum. One of the result of these changed trends was the use of apparatuses. An additional and chief whirling point in his career was the war time. At that time he got trapped in Britain because of war. During that time medical gymnastics emerged as a popular trend. Joseph Pilates also started instructing corrective exercise.

The theme line of Pilates as a fitness instrument is that the powerhouse of human body is the center of the human body. So this technique is exclusively focuses on the postural muscles, to regain a perfect posture. The apparatus used in different sessions, the Allegro Reformer, uses straps, springs, and a stirring carriage to provide for a variety of exercises and to create spatial and body awareness. Pilates is a scheme for attaining the body awareness. Having a firm belief in and having the determination to get results with Pilate's scheme will revolutionize your entire life, the mode of your feeling your own appearance will change altogether

Return to Life through Contrology

Joseph H. Pilates spent a major portion of his life in United States a and made major developments upon his research work there, Therefore United States became the major hub for the progress and popularity of this technique. It is largely being followed in the United States

Although the technique has become renowned all over the world as "Pilates" because of the unprecedented contribution of its inventor, yet the original term coined by the pioneer was Contrology, from the combination of control and logia (being of Greek origin)

In his book Joseph Pilates proposed that this scheme of exercise is basically an art of highly controlled and calculate movements, which, when properly administrated, will have a feeling of a workout, rather than some imposed kind of therapy. owed to constant practicing Pilates retains the ability to aid in getting flexibility, control, strength, develops control and endurance in the entire body and posture. It entails a prominence to breathing, alignment, coordination, and development of a strapping <u>powerhouse</u> and balance. This scheme of exercise brings out for different exercises to be adapted in a variant range of toughness, from commencement to complex or to any other level. The exercise pattern may also alter or vary depending on the personalized goals of practitioner and the choice of instructors.

Pilates had a strong belief that mental strength and physical health are highly and critically dependent on one another.

The mechanical aspects of "Pilates

Joseph Pilates being the inventor of this technique was not only a gymnast. he was also a scientist as well as a, mechanical genius This aided him to accompany his method by a set of useful equipment which he denoted as "apparatus" .The Apparatus acted as an aid to help pick up the pace or the entire process of body alignment, strengthening, stretching, and increased core strength. The best-known and most popular piece today, Reformer, was in the beginning designated as the Universal Reformer, rightly designated for reforming the body universally. As more and more progress HAS Underwent in the flied of Pilates, there has developed a full array of accessories and equipment. This includes the Pedi-Pole, Wunda Chair, Cadillac, High "Electric" Chair, Ladder Barrel and Spine Corrector.

Publications of Joseph Pilates:

- ✓ Your Health: A Corrective System of Exercising (1934)

- ✓ Return to Life Through Contrology (1945)

Modern Pilates embraces both the traditional approach of Pilates, as well as the modern additions in the scheme. The classical approach to Pilates is based on the original and unedited work of Joseph Pilates, the legend; whereas the current versions are based on slight alterations and modifications, made mostly by first generation students. But most of the people are of the view that this mixture of new and old has largely benefited the field and it has expanded the scope of Pilates from being a mere exercise to a whole therapeutic approach. So this addition has benefited a lot for all the practitioners, in various fields, and also put great emphasis for the need of physical health.

At the time when it was first introduced, Pilates technique was confined to specialized surroundings like studios and Pilates center, but as the benefits of Pilates have outburst at an exponential rate, the facility has now been adopted by various gyms, exercise centers and physiotherapy rooms .The major reason for this diversity in the available spaces for Pilates, can easily be accounted for its highly influential effects and far reaching benefits. Many of the physical instructors are modifying this technique along with their own ways of exercise and physical art. This has made the field of Pilates, a greatly enriched field, in which every new day brings a lot of diversity and new techniques. All over the world people now consider it as more of a therapeutic technique, which is bestowing health and rigor all over the world to millions of people who were hopeless after some ailment or their distorted body type.

Chapter 3:
The Astounding Effects of Pilates

Fitness is the first mandatory for contentment and joy. A common belief about the nature of physical fitness is the accomplishment and continuation of a consistently maintained body with an active mind, which entails the capability of undergoing all tasks with promptness and diligence. To attain the premier success, within the boundaries of one's capacities, in all domains and arenas of life, the preceding significance must be given to get healthier and developed body systems. Once physical rigor is established, it will without human intervention overlay the system towards mental zest and intelligence.

But all this is easy to write and say. Once you start implementing this, you will find a lot many hindrances. Among the supreme challenges is to keep streamlined while being in this challenging world, where everything is hard to achieve. The work pressures, the family demands and the individual needs, all sum up to make the life more messy and challenging. In all this one forgets to think and hover upon his own individual being. Most of the time we think that the last priority we think of, is ourselves. We assume it wrongly that our responsibility is to thrive in all fields of life, leaving behind all necessities of our own health. But in this busy scheduled life, we forget that vigor is foreseeable and remote, despite of all financial resources. Once gone, health needs excessive efforts to be restored.

Physical fitness is both a dilemma and a blessing. It is a kind of state which can never be achieved through heavy investments or by ere thinking. It demands for full exertion and efforts. The results are always twofold. Higher the rate of exertion, definitely higher will be the benefits achieved. But the modern system of human civilization has ruined this need of human being, by engaging it in a number of irrelevant and disastrous tasks, including increased reliance on technology and robotic inventions. Although fiscally one may be mountaineering the ladders of triumph, but the health arena of one's life may fall insolvent. So balancing both sides of the pivot is the key for life, eventually one can be labeled as the real victorious person. If an individual is quite successful in the work life, but he has ruined his health and body, he cannot be labeled as a successful man because he has opted for one, among the two most crucial aspects of life,

Among all these panics and challenges, Pilates has emerged as a major revolutionary step. Among a number of different useful aspects of Pilates, some of them are reflected and discussed below:

➢ For weight loss:

One of the major disasters created by this challenging life is the life routines which ultimately make the human body fatty and overweight. Overweight induces a number of various physical issues which can retain for longer periods, ultimately leading to disasters in human health. Pilates is miraculous for weight loss. The systematic procedures and techniques of Pilates lead towards burning of fat that will assist in making the body slimmed and trimmed, within no time. But the key to triumph is the consistency in the routines and practicing of Pilates. This scheme of body exercise help you monitor your body, modify your breathing patterns, so that all these functions of human body can be changed into an efficient and highly effective body system. Most of the Pilates schemes which are aimed for body weight loss denote the stretching exercises.

➢ For dancers

Pilates is not only for curative purposes, meaning that it is not only a technique for the curative purposes. It is not for all those who have ruined their body postures and shape, it can also help a lot many who are involved in a number of stretching professions or other activities which involve excessive physical outputs. Among these professionals, one of the largest groups involves dancers. Dancers are therapists who use their body language to convey their art. They cannot afford even a minimum sort of body disturbances. Moreover, a number of Pilate's techniques involve the postures which ultimately lead to highly flexible body organs, so it aid in using the body more effectively by the dancers. Various dancers have reported that they have experienced a wide appreciation because of changed body reflexive due to Pilates.

➢ During pregnancy

Many women think that they are cannot exert much physical efforts if they have got pregnant. Pregnancy does not denote physical statistic. It must be accompanied with healthy routines and living patterns. Pilates is a distinctive workout scheme which can pose a number of techniques for pregnant ladies, which will not only lend a hand to them for retaining their body shapes but will also aid in progressive development of the baby's body. Although pregnancy needs excessive monitoring for body, yet it does not demand that all the physical activity must be stopped immediately after getting the good news. The whole period of pregnancy must be engaged in a way that it becomes productive for the health and physique, not a burden. Pilates introduces some basic regimes of body and leg movement for all ladies who are having these issues and help them cater their pregnancy in a better way. If the women start it form the initial stage to last stage she will definitely enjoy an overwhelmingly secure and sound pregnancy without any complications.

➢ For belly fat

Some specific issues addressed by Pilates also include the belly fat issues. Any excessive fat deposit or lipoid-deposit is easily manageable by some modified techniques of Pilates, which help in calorie burning and fat dissolution. Many of the thinkers hold the analysis that belly fat reduction demands for a consistent approach towards following a regular scheme. Belly fat reduction is considered as one of the major challenges as well as a hindrance towards slim and trim body. Many of the Pilates techniques have been specially modified, to help a large number of people, who are facing a downturn in their body. The reason for this downturn is the increased fat on their belly. It also hits the body and the personality charisma. No one likes to be recognized by a loose tummy. So Pilates can help everyone start an energetic and charismatic life by trimming the belly and making all the muscles healthy strong and still attractive.

➢ For back pain

One of the key reasons for back ache is the distorted body postures. These postures are usually induced by unhealthy sitting postures and uncomfortable sitting plan. Moreover back pain can be because of higher tendency towards obesity and the tendency of being overweight. All these basic reasons can contribute towards the highly painful condition of back ache. Pilates is aimed at not only curing back ache nut also preventing it in all those, who have not encountered it. The stretching exercises and the postures introduced by Pilates help in strengthen of spinal cord and the vertebrae so that it can maintain the back strength and avoid all the reasons effectively. Back ache has been reported to be one of the major reasons of distorted body shapes, so eradicating it form the basic level is highly crucial.

> ### For abs

Another misconception about Pilate's method is that it is only a way of correcting the posture, body movements and breathing patterns. Many people are devoid of the information that Pilates is also for all those who want to build up a muscular body. Abs building is another miracle of Pilate's scheme of exercise. Although the scheme and pattern of exercise will be quite transformed for abs building, yet Pilates is not devoid of these kinds of techniques which are helpful for body builders and all those who are interested in muscle formation. Many people have been successful in building and sustain their abs because they have consistently followed Pilate's scheme.